Aline Brum
Aline Belletti
Laura Perim

The Dynamics of Nursing Practice

Aline Brum
Aline Belletti
Laura Perim

The Dynamics of Nursing Practice

Reflections on Practice

ScienciaScripts

Imprint

Cover image: www.ingimage.com

This book is a translation from the original published under ISBN 978-3-639-61487-9.

Publisher:
Sciencia Scripts
is a trademark of
Dodo Books Indian Ocean Ltd. and OmniScriptum S.R.L publishing group

120 High Road, East Finchley, London, N2 9ED, United Kingdom
Str. Armeneasca 28/1, office 1, Chisinau MD-2012, Republic of Moldova, Europe
Printed at: see last page
ISBN: 978-620-6-46060-2

The Dynamics of Nursing Practice

SUMMARY

1. REFLECTING ON THE DYNAMIC NATURE OF NURSES' WORK

Nursing is characterised as a science that works with individuals and communities, planning and carrying out actions that permeate care. In Brazil, the profession is carried out by nursing assistants, nursing technicians and nurses, professionals with different training and functions within the same area. In Brazil, the profession is exercised by nursing assistants, nursing technicians and nurses, professionals with different training and functions within the same area (SOUSA et al, 2017).

The central focus of nursing work is caring for human beings, in all their complexity, and it is on this care that nursing produces knowledge and technologies to support its disciplinary field and which underpins its profession (RAMOS, PIRES and BERTONCINIL, 2013).

The work of nurses, according to Leopardi, Gelbeck and Ramos, 2012, is characterised by four dimensions: direct care for individuals or groups, from conception to death; educational dimensions, consisting of professional training processes, continuing education and health education with the user; administrative/managerial dimensions, coordinating and organising nursing work and participating in health care management; investigative dimensions, producing knowledge to support and guide the processes of care, management and health education.

According to Junior and Matsuda (2012), nurses' activities are based on various interconnected actions that are structured on the basis of care, administrative/managerial, investigative and educational practices. In practice, these actions are carried out between the components of the nursing team, with the nurse remaining the articulating and integrating link in the work of nursing as a whole. A striking feature of nurses' work is the fact that it includes care, administrative/managerial, teaching and research activities, carried out in an interdependent manner (JUNIOR E MATSUDA, 2012).

The structuring of the health network, which is still centred on procedures and places too much value on medical knowledge, has brought into question the way in which comprehensive care has taken place in the various devices of the health system. Nurses work as team members in a multidisciplinary team, and in this sense, the way in which their actions are carried out must be aimed at meeting the health needs of individuals and the community. As part of this context, the nurse's management practice includes coordination, supervision and evaluation actions, produced in the processes of guidance, dialogue and negotiation between the team, users and families (SOUSA, AUED, GUIMARAES, 2018).

According to Hausmann and Peduzzi, 2017, care management is interpreted as the clearest expression of good nursing practice, where there is articulation between the managerial and care dimensions to meet the care needs of patients and at the same time of the nursing team and the institution. The realisation of good practice in nurses' actions permeates scientific knowledge, planning, management, performance and evaluation of the established goals. This set of dimensions is anchored in humanisation and patient safety.

Attention, concentration and memory can be impaired due to the mental rumination of problems and excessive preoccupation with personal problems, difficulties in maintaining social contacts and suicidal ideas, which can cause reduced quality of life, increased absenteeism from work, reduced quality of care and ultimately suicide (BARSOSA et al, 2017).

Various factors influence the suffering of nursing professionals, such as work overload, excessive working hours, overcrowded care units, devaluation of the profession, constant work with suffering and pain, among others. Nursing demands attention and a more humane approach to nursing professionals is needed.

REFERENCES: Sousa SM, Aued GK, Bernardino E, Guimaraes MP. The role of nurses in a functional unit management model In: Vale EG, Peruzzo SA, Felli VEA. (org). Nursing Update Programme. Management: cycle 4. Porto Alegre: Artmed; 2018.p.77-104.

JUNIOR, J.A.B; MATSUDA, L.H.G. O enfermeiro no gerenciamento à qualidade em Serviço Hospitalar de Emergência: revisão integrativa da literatura. Rev Gaúcha Enferm, Porto Alegre (RS) 2012 Dec;32(4):797-806. Available at: <http://www.scielo.br/scielo.php?script=sciarttext&pid=S1983-14472011000400022>. Accessed on: 20 June 2019.

LEOPARDI, MT; GELBECKE, FL; RAMOS, FRS. Care: work objective or epistemological object of nursing? Texto e Contexto Enfermagem, 2012; 10(1): 32 - 49.

Sousa SM, Bernardino E, Crozeta K, Peres AM, Lacerda MR. Integrality of care: challenges for the nurse practice. Rev Bras Enferm. 2017;70(3):504-10. Available at:

<http://www.scielo.br/scielo.php?script=sciarttext&pid=S0034-71672017000300504>. Accessed on: 25 July 2019.

2. Barbosa, Khivia Kiss Silva; Vieira, Kay Francis Leal; Alves, Estela Rodrigues Paiva; Virgínio, Nereide Andrade. **DEPRESSIVE SYMPTOMS AND SUICIDAL IDEATION IN HOSPITAL NURSES AND DOCTORS.** Available at: <https://periodicos.ufsm.br/reufsm/article/view/5910/pdf> Accessed on: 25 May 2019

2. POLITICAL ADVOCACY BY NURSES IN THE FACE OF POWER

Aline Belletti Figueira

SUMMARY

The aim was to reflect on the process of political advocacy by nurses in the face of power relations. To this end, a reflective approach was adopted, based on a theoretical study of the concept of political advocacy by nurses in the face of power relations. Through critical awareness, nurses seek knowledge in order to interact in power relations, with the possibility of taking action in political advocacy in defence of users with regard to improvements in health conditions and quality of life. By enabling nurses to develop skills to better act in defence of users, with the construction of links in interactions, with the aim of qualifying this work. The conclusion is that the environment in which nurses work is a preponderant factor in the development of relational skills to better advocate. Ethical commitment to the profession means that nurses are able to carry out political advocacy with excellence to benefit as many people as possible.

Keywords: Political advocacy; Nursing; Power.

1. INTRODUCTION

Over the years, nurses have emerged as professionals who specialise in caring for human beings at different points in their lives, developing their work through constant interaction with the individuals who need it. To this end, they qualify their profession through in-depth studies on care, guided by ethics and morality in their relationships with other nurses, other health professionals and users.

Allied to disease prevention, health promotion, rehabilitation according to needs and especially in situations of defence of the patient/user when they are not in a position to decide on their health, this is perceived as an act of defence, of advocacy. According to the World Health Organization (WHO)[1] health advocacy is the combination of individual and social actions aimed at gaining support, political commitment, social acceptance and systems support for a particular health goal or programme, through various interpersonal means, institutions and the media, going beyond legal advocacy proper[1] .

It doesn't just concern the relationship between user and nurse, but is a triad: nurses, users and other people in the healthcare environment. Therefore, as well as carrying out their activities with excellence, nurses must have direct contact with situations that lead them to act as political agents, seeking changes in defence of users and the community 2.

Since user advocacy sheds light on issues of social justice, whether individual or collective, to advocate at the social level for significant changes related to people's well-being[3] . Therefore, the practice of health advocacy focuses on the defence of human rights and tends to create conditions for autonomy, equality and justice in social relations, as well as equal access to opportunities for all 4.

In this practice, nurses use evidence and experience from their actions with a more effective impact at both local and international level to improve health care and strengthen their autonomy 5. We realise that the more knowledge and responsibility nurses have, the better their competence to intervene in political advocacy.

In defence, political advocacy stands out as an action aimed at promoting social justice and the health of individuals, communities and populations. As such, it has a direct influence on reducing health inequalities and socio-environmental risk conditions, such as poor access to high-quality care, improved health quality, poverty reduction, precarious housing, among others 6.

In addition, interactions with different institutions and organisations provide nurses with the means to be health advocates, with the possibility of making significant changes to people's quality of life. According to Foucalt (1991), the subject relates to the world based on relations of power and knowledge, and the neutrality of actions does not exist[(7)] . Therefore, anyone can exercise power and what will determine this is each person's ability to produce knowledge and use it positively in their favour.

The aim of this article is to reflect on the process of political advocacy by nurses in the face of power relations. Realising the need for proactive action by nurses to promote quality of life for human beings, and seeing the importance of nurses' political advocacy for users in improving health care, as well as the need to understand the process of political advocacy by nurses in the face of power relations, **justifies** this study.

The relevance of this work lies in the fact that nurses perceive political advocacy as a necessary action to promote direct care for a large number of people in different life contexts. With emphasis on the **research problem**, which is: How does the process of political advocacy by nurses occur in the face of power relations?

2. METHODOLOGY

A reflection was made on the basis of an in-depth study of the literature in various national and international databases on the subject of "Political advocacy in nursing in the face of power relations". The author who served as the basis for reflection was Michel Foucault, in particular his writings on power relations, applied to the process of political advocacy by nurses.

The search was carried out between March and July 2016. The development of this study took place in two stages. The first involved choosing the philosopher to reflect on.

The second step was to search for articles in different national and international databases using the following descriptors: Political Advocacy; Nursing; Power; with the aim of greater immersion, as this would allow an in-depth analysis of the selected texts identified for this assertion.

NURSING AND POLITICAL ACTION: a historical review

With the Brazilian Health Reform, they began to see health as a social and political issue to be addressed in different public spaces 9. Then, in the new Constitution of the Republic, promulgated in 1988, the State became responsible for guaranteeing the right to comprehensive health for all Brazilian citizens, through the creation of a system of universal and equal access, with actions aimed at promoting, protecting and recovering health, the Unified Health System (SUS)[10] . Participatory management was defined as an important innovation in national health 1[1] .

In this way, nursing as an integral part of the health system and a professional that is part of the participatory management of the SUS is directly involved in creating a future built on responsibility and sustainability, as well as requiring the professional's critical awareness of health care in different contexts in order to promote better care 2.

Therefore, care, taken as the object of nursing knowledge and practice, is configured as an act carried out in the field of action with the aim of promoting and maintaining health, the environment, comfort and well-being. In the light of this paradigm, people need to be present in the care process, participate, create and recreate ways of thinking and acting in favour of health. This care requires social participation, citizen awareness, reflection and action so that it actually takes place [12]

In the meantime, nursing is a dynamic social profession, subject to constant transformation and the incorporation of reflections and actions on new issues/problems guided by the ethical principle of maintaining or restoring dignity in the different areas of life. To do this, it needs to develop a comprehensive and interactive view of social and health issues, in line with the complexity and pluralities of today's society[13] .

Their work shows a long history of mobilisation to address political issues related to users. These actions often have a direct influence on the political choices made by governments to improve the health and well-being of the population [14]

In this way, it participates in programmes and services for specific groups aimed at reducing inequalities in health, with engagement in political actions in order to promote the development of effective policies, with the ability to deal with diversities / inequalities in health and thus identify effective interventions through investigative studies that address this context [15]

In addition, understanding complex issues in public policy requires attention to intervention networks that go beyond local, national and international borders, with the interaction of ideologies, interests, commodities and power dynamics [14]

Thus, health in local, national and global contexts will benefit from nurses' political vision, given the strength of the profession and the value of their work in society. By strengthening influences in nursing, teaching and working in public policy, they share experiences and knowledge with a large number of people, as well as improving their knowledge of issues related to care [5].

In this way, nurses get to know and experience users' conditions directly, acquiring and organising resources for the best care. They also gain confidence and competence in their work, as they are able to perceive users' needs, increasing their political power to defend the population's health. [14]

Thus, problem-solving and health gains are more likely to occur with the union of various sectors (government, health staff, nursing in particular, the community, among others) in bringing health knowledge directly related to the target populations. In addition to viewing nursing as a profession with a great capacity for interaction, which often makes them the biggest providers of health and the first to recognise health problems and the need for policy changes to address related issues[14] .

The political role is therefore seen as an extension of the idea of health advocacy, since advocating for health requires articulation in defence of something, a population or groups, with constant reflection on the principles of health promotion. Thus, through the concept of advocacy, the "political role" stands out as one of the main means, one of the main strategies for exercising advocacy by nurses [16]

NURSING IN POLITICAL ADVOCACY

The act of advocating requires nurses to have prior knowledge and skills, personal characteristics of leadership and proactivity, as well as the unity of the multidisciplinary team, a good level of communication, a good relationship with users and their families and recognition of their needs and desires, which means greater commitment/involvement in advocacy. [16]

Experiences of advocacy will arise from these interactions, since multiple environments make up human life and have a direct influence on individuals' behaviour and ethical interactions. The perception of individual and collective needs in these exchanges stands out [18]

Working from the perspective of political advocacy by social actors takes place in the validation of collective and individual rights, in the pursuit of basic health rights that are not guaranteed by law or are not respected by the state, through political strategies, with the aim of influencing decision-making by the authorities. [19]

Therefore, the characteristics of professionals will have a direct and positive influence on the practice of law, such as when they show greater confidence in their professional value, knowledge and responsibility[18] .

In this way, advocacy is a fundamental skill for nurses to develop the political role and guidelines of health promotion as a practice for active citizenship and to give continuity and sustainability to their actions 20.

It is worth emphasising that political advocacy helps people to obtain quality services, benefits and unpromoted rights that improve their quality of life. Thus, they are interventions aimed at changes in health policies in institutions, communities and government that advocate improvements in the well-being of a significant number of users in a community[21] . It's an opportunity for nurses to "advocate" for a larger number of people.

Therefore, they need to define priorities and urgencies related to patients' unfulfilled rights, as well as discussing these priorities with the other participants. Defining them helps nurses to broaden their range of actions and set clearer objectives in line with needs[14] .

In addition, political advocacy has the potential to prevent user problems related to violation of ethical rights, poor quality of services, lack of cultural responsiveness, lack of preventive care, expensive treatments, inability to solve mental health problems, inability to provide care to families and the community[21] ,2 .[2]

In this way, health promotion based on political advocacy by nurses is expressed in the actions of organised groups and/or individuals who seek health, intervening in their way of living and surviving[14] . These actions will be reflected in the critical awareness of nurses and in their power as knowledge practitioners.

NURSING AND THE EXERCISE OF POWER: Possibilities for political advocacy

Changes in power relations are concrete realities for professional nurses who seek to build forms of resistance that go beyond simply accepting the context as it is. In order to do this, they need to have a level of perception that allows them to understand the fine lines that power runs through the life of each nurse, in their multiple relationships, promoting a moral stance that is consistent with the practice to be carried out, which is caring for human beings[2] 3,[24] .

Thus, nurses, as professionals at the forefront of political advocacy, need to constantly increase their awareness of their power in society, in order to act both in defence of their profession and in defence of the rights of citizens/users in health care[16] From this perspective, the knowledge needed to act in political advocacy changes according to the progress of power relations, since there is no neutrality in the production of knowledge, there will always be power relations in a power/knowledge binary. In this relationship, whoever holds the knowledge assumes a higher position; as well as realising that the relationships are cyclical, circular, with some holding power at times and others at others, since it changes according to the interactions between the different[24] .

The ethics of self-care also come to the fore in this exercise of the profession as the way in which the individual is constituted as the subject of their own actions, their responsibilities in direct relation to their actions towards others[25] Therefore, nurses must provide excellent care that reaches as many people as possible with the consequent improvement of health in a global context.

It is important in these interrelationships to realise the subjectivities involved and, even more so, to take on the responsibility of advocating on their behalf as an important challenge in the profession.

Subjectivity in these exchanges will always be unfinished and constantly being reformulated. It is both process and product. Process as it is constructed, it requires changes, adaptations in search of new subjectivations and as a product it refers to the unique and unfinished subject in this environment 24. It will be individual and will depend on the experiences and knowledge of those involved.

There is no power relationship without resistance, without the possibility of an inversion in the intensity of power relations. Thus, every power relationship implies at least the desire to fight, to confront, which seeks to establish a new power relationship, transforming barriers through resistance strategies [23,25]. The subject is constituted at the intersection of knowledge/power [26].

3. CONCLUSION

In the end, we realise that the contribution of this study goes beyond encouraging nurses to take political advocacy actions in the face of power relations. It reinforces the professional's potential to interact in different relationships with a broader knowledge of health issues, a foundation that needs to be constantly developed in order to promote health and guarantee the quality of life of those involved.

In addition, the professional's knowledge of their potential for defence and communication with other people in their workplaces allows them to constantly re-evaluate their work process, with a view to improving care and, consequently, improving the health of their populations.

Thus, nurses committed to political advocacy will be in a position to intervene positively to improve the health of individuals, communities, nationally and internationally, reaching a greater number of people. Therefore, changes in the perspective of care will promote new ways of perceiving health, through nursing with a broader vision, capable of perceiving and respecting the different environments in which it operates.

REFERENCES

1. World Health Organisation. Advocacy Strategies for Health and Development: **Development Communication in Action**. Geneva: WHO, 1995.

2. Ventura CAA et al. Nursing's alliance with users in the defence of the SUS. **Rev. Bras. Enferm.** 2012;65(6):893-8. Available at: http://www.scielo.br/scielo.php?script=sciarttext&pid=S0034- 71672012000600002. Accessed on 20 September 2018.

3. Hanks RG. Social Advocacy: A Call for Nursing Action. **Pastoral Psychology.** 2013;62(2):163-73.

4. Pavlish C; Ho A; Rounkle A. Health and human rights advocacy: perspectives from a Rwandan refugee camp. **Nursing Ethics**. 2012;19(4):538- 49. Available at : www.ncbi.nlm.nih.gov/pubmed/22496055. Accessed 25 September 2018.

5. Shamiami J. The role of nursing in health care. **Rev Bras Enferm**. 2014;67(6):869-70. Disponívelem: <http://www.scielo.br/pdf/reben/v67n6/pt 0034-7167-reben-67-06-0867.pdf > Accessed on 27 July 2018.

6. Taylor, Melissa RS. Impact of Advocacy Initiatives on Nurses' Motivation to Sustain Momentum in Public Policy Advocacy. **Journal of Professional Nursing**. 2016;32(3): 235-45. Available at: www.ncbi.nlm.nih.gov/pubmed/27216131. Accessed 16 December 2018.

7. Foucault, M., Gordon, C., Miller, P., Burchell, G. The Foucault effect: studies in governmentality: with two lectures by and an interview with Michel Foucault. Harvester Wheatsheaf, 1991.

8. Paim J et al. Health in Brazil. The Brazilian health system: history, advances and challenges. **Veja**. 2012;6736(11):60054-8.

9. Nascimento MS; Nascimento MAA. Nurse practice in the Family Health Programme: the interface of health surveillance versus programmatic health actions. **Cienc. Saúde Colet**. 2005;10(2):333-45. Available at:http://www.scielo.br/scielo.php?script=sciarttext&pid=S1413-81232005000200011 >. Accessed on 25 January 2019.

10. Junior AP; Junior LC. Public health policies in Brazil. **Rev, Espaço for Health**. 2006. Available at: www.unasus.unifesp.br/biblioteca virtual/esf/1/modulopolitical-manager/Unit 4. pdf. Accessed on 20 October 2018.

11. Foucalt, M. Truth and subjectivity. **Journal of communication and language**. Lisbon. 1993;19(1):203-23.

12. Ferreira MA. The classic and the emerging: challenges of production, of dissemination and utilisation of nursing knowledge. **Rev. Bras. Enferm.** 2013;66(n. spe):45-50. Available at: http://www.scielo.br/scielo.php?script=sciarttext&pid=S0034- 71672013000700006. Accessed on 20 October 2018.

13. Zobolo ELCP; Schveitzer MC. Nursing values as a practice social: a qualitative meta-synthesis. **Revista Latino-Americana de Enfermagem**. 2013;21(3):695-703. Available at : http://www.scielo.br/pdf/rlae/v21n3/pt 0104-1169-rlae-21-03-0695.pdf. Accessed on 22 November 2018.

14. MacDonald JA et al. Priority setting and policy advocacy by nursing associations: A scoping review and implications using a socio-ecological whole systems lens. **Health Policy**. 2012; 107(1):31-43.

15. Cohen BE; Reutter L. Development of the role of public health nurses in addressing child and family poverty: a framework for action. **Journal of**

AdvancedNursing. 2007;60(1):96-107. Available at: www.ncbi.nlm.nih.gov/pubmed/17459126. Accessed 21 September 2018.

16. Gandra EC. **The defence of health and the political action of nurses: competences for health promotion in professional training**. 2014. Doctoral thesis. Federal University of Minas Gerais. School of Nursing.

17. Hanks RG. The medical-surgical nurse perspective of advocate role. **Nursing Forum**. 2010;45(2):97-107.

18. Negarandeh R. et al. Patient advocacy: barriers and facilitators. **BMC Nursing.** 2006;5(3):1-8.

19. Brito CM. Health advocacy and non-governmental organisations in the Federal District. **Cadernos Ibero-Americanos de Derecho Sanitario.** 2014;2(1):22-39.

20. Canel RC; Castro CGJ. Health advocacy as a strategy for health promotion. **Revista de Direito Sanitário.** 2008;9(1):74-85.

21. Jansson BS et al. Validation of the Policy Advocacy Engagement Scale for frontline healthcare professionals. **Nursing Ethics**. 2015;0969733015603443.

22. Schluter J et al. Nurses' moral sensitivity and hospital ethical climate: a literature review. **Nursing Ethics**. 2008;15(3):304-21.

23. Tomaschewski-Barlem JG et al. How should nurses practise patient advocacy in the hospital context? A foucaltian perspective. **Texto & Contexto-Enfermagem**. 2016;25(1). Disponívelem : http://www.scielo.br/scielo.php?pid=S0104-07072016000100308&script=sciarttext&tlng=en. Accessed on 08 January 2019.

24. Foucault M. **Microfísica do poder**. 26ª ed. Rio de Janeiro (RJ): Edições Graal; 2008.

25. Foucalt M. Truth, power and the self. In: Foucalt M. **Ditos e Escritos** V: ética, sexualidade e política. Rio de Janeiro: Forense Universitária, 2004.

26. Foucault, M. (1985). History of Sexuality III: **The Care of** the **Self** (M. T. C. Albuquerque, transl.). Rio de Janeiro: Graal.

3. A reflection on the construction of the concept of health

Laura Fontoura Perim, Aline Neutzling Brum, Juliane Scarton, Jeferson Ventura, Saul Ferraz de Paula

1. INTRODUCTION

The social, economic and technological changes of recent years have led to significant transformations in the way work is organised and also in the types of services provided to the population, as well as in the way human beings think, do and live, impacting on ways of understanding health.

According to Batistella, 2007, separating the health-disease binomial has become a necessary and emerging practice nowadays, unlike disease, in relation to health it is difficult to propose a common sense definition throughout history. The trajectory of humanity is made up of the development and construction of the concept of health over time, influenced by the characteristics of each period.

Health, despite being a field of concern and arousing research interest throughout its history, was given a new connotation in the Brazilian Federal Constitution of 1988. In Article 196 of the Constitution, health came to be understood as a right of all and a duty of the state, provided through social and economic policies to reduce the risk of disease and illness, as well as universal and equal access to actions and services, aimed at promoting, protecting and recovering the health of users (BRASIL, 2003). This broad definition of health is still with us today and drives our research and investigations into this subject.

According to Batistella, 2017, the view of health as the absence of disease is widespread in common sense, but it is not restricted to this dimension of knowledge. Studies and research are delving deeper into theorising an expanded concept of health that relates the individual and their biological and psychological/social dimensions to the environment they are in and their interaction with it.

Individuals are involved in the dynamics of their relationships and interaction with the elements that make up their reality, where these elements, which contribute directly to their health condition, make it possible for changes to be built on the basis of the individual and the community. From this perspective, it can be seen that individuals can improve their condition and achieve a better quality of life when they contribute to the context in which they live, both in terms of the health institutions and services available, as well as the other aspects that make up their reality (WEYCAMP, 2015).

Health is presented as the sum of the dynamic balance that brings together the physical, psychological, sociocultural and spiritual dimensions of the human being, and their interactions with the environment. In this view, health can be defined as a subjective and particular experience, something that can be expressed individually, known intuitively, but never described collectively or quantified (SIQUEIRA et al , 2018).

Health and illness have always been part of the reality of health services and institutions, as well as human perception. According to Weycamp, 2015, throughout human history, health has suffered cultural, economic, political and educational influences, contributing to the formation of society and leading to innovation in different approaches to health issues.

The justification for this work makes it necessary to reflect on and discuss the concept of health today. The perception of current health needs guides the reflection based on readings that work on the proposed theme, anchored by the professional experience and experiences that each author carries.

2. OBJECTIVE

The aim is to reflect on and discuss the construction of the concept of health.

3. METHODOLOGY

This is a study of theoretical and physiological reflection. The discussion is based on one axis: the construction of the concept of health based on the proposed readings and discussions in the classroom and with the help of alternative literature.

This was followed by a critical-analytical reading of the texts in order to select the most significant approaches to health concepts.

4. RESULTS

After understanding and reading, the definition is that health is related to how each individual interacts with life events, because the concept of a health need does not impact on all people in the same way. Health is a process of balance between being well and being well according to each person's lifestyle. What characterises health is the ability of human beings to adapt to their environment. The need for health implies a person's relationship with the external environment and their own internal conditions.

FIGURE 1 - ELABORATION OF THE CONCEPT OF HEALTH

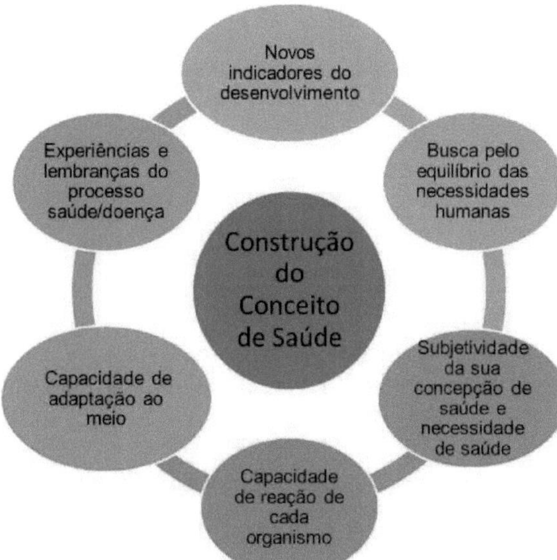

Source: Prepared from the theoretical framework. Organised by PERIM, 2019.

5. DISCUSSION

With the creation of the Unified Health System (SUS), health came to be understood as a right of citizenship and a duty of the state. Based on the principles of universality, equity and comprehensiveness and the guidelines of decentralisation, regionalisation and community participation, the SUS reaffirms health as a value and a fundamental human right, legitimised by social justice (BRASIL, 1986). This expanded concept of health ensures that all citizens can exercise their social and individual rights.

Capra (2006) stresses the importance of analysing health as a multidimensional process, subject to transformation, by analysing the relationships between physical, biological, socio-cultural, economic, psychological and spiritual elements with the individual and the community. The end product of this interaction results in new health needs.

The focus on health conditions and quality of life are in contrast to one's own reading of the world and of oneself in that world. The baggage that each person brings with experiences and memories of the health/disease process, experienced throughout life, influences lifestyle changes in both positive and negative ways.

According to Camargo, 2015, the understanding of the world is based on the concept of the search for happiness, influencing the health-disease process through small achievements. The concept of a small health need doesn't impact on everyone in the same way, but living through this experience can make people aware of the need to change their lifestyle in order to achieve healthy and active ageing.

The fear of the unknown is common and being able to share it with someone is a way of alleviating it (CAMARGO, 2015). Understanding the condition of health needs brings together people who are going through the same difficulties. According to Camargo, 2015, chronic suffering transforms the joy of small things and small achievements into learning. Appreciation of health conditions accompanies the chronically ill, impacting on their reading of the world.

Health is considered an absolute model, a normative concept that defines an ideal type of organic structure and behaviour. Health goes beyond the norm that defines the momentary normal, tolerating infractions of the usual norm and instituting a new regulation. Health is related to how each individual interacts with life events.

Canguilhen's 2012 interpretation of health is in line with the process in which an organism suffers normative losses, but its ability to adapt to new norms reconstitutes the initial state or adapts it to a new reality. Illness differs from health, the pathological from the normal. To master illness is to understand its relationship with the normal state that the living person wishes to restore. The threat of illness is one of the elements that condition health.

What characterises health is the human being's ability to adapt to the environment in which they find themselves, especially the influence that external actions can have on the organism. According to Canguilhen, 2012, health is a guide that regulates the possibilities of reaction. An organism that feels healthy is one that is not only adapted to the environment and its demands, but is also capable of following the new norms of life. Analysing that man needs to adapt to the environment in which he lives reinforces the importance of working on health actions with a focus on prevention. By knowing each person's risk factors, it becomes effective to draw up a line of individual care, but with an eye on priority groups.

Canguilhem, 2012 states that health implies being able to get sick and get out of the pathological state. In other words, health is understood by reference to the possibility of facing new situations, the margin of tolerance or security that each person has to face and overcome the infidelities of the environment, or even a regulatory guide for each organism's reaction possibilities. This approach reinforces the fact that the idea of health as the absence of disease has been broadened by the perspective of health as the possibility of becoming ill.

The pathological fact as an alteration of the normal state can only be defined as and learnt as an organic totality (CANGUILHEM, 2012). We can understand that no illness carries with it only negative feelings, but rather a new normative of the human being. The possibility of an organism adapting is to live a new life, thus constructing new norms and ways of creating adjustments with this environment and we can interpret that life does not fit into pre-established norms.

The experience of being alive includes the experience of becoming ill, so we believe that healing practices are guided by the notion of health and not just the restoration of illness.

In order to understand the complexity that surrounds health, it is necessary to evaluate the multiplicity of elements and processes that directly and indirectly influence its consolidation. This idea demonstrates that the expanded concept of health and the new model of care that results from it trigger transformations in user care (WEYCAMP, 2015). In this line of thought, it is worth noting that the implementation of home care services allows actions to be optimised in the home, close to the reality of each user.

Understanding care actions through home care makes it easier for professionals to plan their actions. It brings prevention and health promotion actions closer to the reality of each context in which the user is inserted. Thus, it is in this context of health actions that the importance of care in an integrated, interdependent and shared way is emphasised, in order to produce knowledge and keep it in constant inter-relationship and cooperation, making it possible for professionals to care for users and their families in their environment/space in an effective and efficient way, strengthening the breadth of the definition of health.

What characterises health is the human being's ability to adapt to the environment in which they find themselves, especially the influence that external actions can have on the organism. According to Canguilhen, health is a guide that regulates the possibilities of reaction. The organism that feels healthy is the one that is not only adapted to the environment and its demands, but is also capable of following the new norms of life. Analysing that man needs to adapt to the environment in which he lives reinforces the importance of working on health actions with a focus on prevention. By knowing each person's risk factors, it becomes effective to draw up a line of individual care, but with an eye on priority groups.

Health can be interpreted as a process that is moulded according to each person's lifestyle. The process of becoming ill is strongly related to environmental, social and cultural factors. Correlating a broad definition of health with Marx's interpretation of the labour process and the process of producing surplus value, we see health as the raw material of a process, with the end product influenced by the determining and conditioning factors in this process, in the labour process it is related to the means of work and in health to habits and lifestyles.

For Marx, a product is a use value, a material from nature adapted to human needs by changing its form. In health, the result of a healthy ageing process is related to the adaptation of human needs in the context in which this being is inserted, favouring or compromising the final result and resulting in different conditions of human survival.

The perception of an expanded concept of health allows us to analyse the whole, but it is becoming increasingly necessary to work on actions more focused on the specific context of each user. The idea of subjectivity as an industrial, machinic nature, i.e. essentially manufactured, modelled, received and consumed (GUATTARI, 2017). Representing the projection of health actions into a mechanised process driven by industrialisation.

Health needs to be interpreted as a process of construction that is the result of a series of agents where the subject is the end and these agents are the process of formation of this subject (GUATTARI, 2017). To the extent that policies take health into account in all these phases of formation, it becomes possible to draw up actions that take into account the health needs of each individual. Corroborating Guattari's idea that we are subjects in the collective sense, policies need to be drawn up based on the user's needs and interaction with the environment in which they find themselves.

According to Left, 2012, quality of life as an objective of sustainable development breaks down the homogeneous parameters of well-being and opens up the possibility of new indicators of human development that articulate the costs of growth with cultural values and the potential of nature. Quality of life is established through the process of re-presenting people's living conditions in relation to their needs and subjective values.

An important issue when analysing quality of life is the individual's perception of their conditions of existence. Health is related to each individual's perception of their condition, cultures and values. Health is influenced by quality of life, behaviour in harmony with the environment, as well as socio-environmental degradation caused by rationality and discounting the future.

Brazil has been undergoing major economic, social and demographic changes, particularly in the last four decades, with significant repercussions on the population's living and working conditions and consequently on their health situation (BRASIL, 2008). Unequal access to health services has an impact on preventive and health promotion actions. The breadth of the national territory characterises a wealth of culture, but impacts on social inequalities and reflects in the diversification of social determinants that impact on the population's health conditions.

According to the Final Report of the National Commission on Social Determinants of Health (CNDSS), the socio-economic, cultural and environmental conditions of a given society, i.e. the more general and distal determinants, generate an economic and social stratification of individuals and population groups, giving them different social positions, which in turn cause health differentials.

We can understand that intervention in the mechanisms of social stratification is one of the most crucial to combating health inequalities, including the need to develop policies that reduce social differences. A second set of policies should seek to reduce the differentials in exposure to risks, taking as an example groups that live in unhealthy housing conditions, work in unsafe environments or are exposed to nutritional deficiencies (BRASIL, 2008).

According to Siqueira et al 2018, we can understand that health is not just the absence of disease, but the search for the balance of human needs anchored in the set of relationships between the elements that make up the ecosystem. Understanding these elements enables health professionals to understand the influence of the individual's interaction with the environment in which they find themselves, from a macro, meso and micro social perspective.

5. FINAL CONSIDERATIONS

It is necessary to understand health as a dynamic, multifactorial and cyclical process. The conceptualisation is constantly changing, influenced by various factors such as politics, the environment, biological and sectoral issues. As professionals involved in the health and illness process, it is the nurse's role to understand the multifaceted nature of this process in order to adapt it to the needs of each individual.

Understanding the concept of health in its various interfaces favours health professionals in building an individual line of care for each individual, as well as understanding public policies.

It is the role of academia to encourage students to develop a broader view of the concept of health, adapting it to the country's diverse realities. Carrying out health actions is in line with understanding the variations in the concept of health, looking at the individual and the community.

References CAMARGO, J.J. **What do you need to be happy?** 1 ed. Porto Alegre, RS:LPM, 2015

CAPRA, F. **O ponto de mutação**. São Paulo, Cultrix, 2006.

CANGUILHEM, G. **The normal and the pathological.** 7ª ed. Rio de Janeiro: Forense

- Universitária, 2012

MARX, K. **Capital**. Critique of political economy. 10 Ed. São Paulo: Difel. Book. I, v.1, 1985. Chap. 5, p.201 - 223.

Ministry of Health. 8th National Health Conference. In: Proceedings of the 8th National Health Conference. Brasília, Rio de Janeiro, DF: The Ministry; 1986.

WEYCAMP, J.M. **Nursing Care for SUS Users in Home Care Services from an Ecosystem Perspective**. Rio Grande, 2015

GUATARRI, F.; ROLINK, S. **Micropolitics - cartographies of desire**. 7th Ed. Revisited. Petrópoles: Editora Vozes; 2005.

BATISTELLA, C. **Contemporary Approaches to the Concept of Health**. Rio de Janeiro: Fiocruz, 2017.

BRAZIL, **The Social Causes of Health Inequities in Brazil**. 2008

LEFT, E. **Saber Ambiental: sustentabilidade, racionalidade, complexidade, poder**. 9th Ed. Petrópoles, RJ: Vozes, 2012.

SIQUEIRA, HCH; THUROW, MRB; PAULA, SP; ZAMBERLAN, C; MEDEIROS, AC; CECAGNO, D; SAMPAIO, A; PERIM, L. The health of the human being from an acositemic perspective. Rev enferm UFPE on line, Recife, 12(2):559-64, Feb., 2018.

Batistella C. The territory and the health-disease process. Rio de Janeiro: FIOCRUZ; 2007.

4. FACTORS THAT TRIGGER DEPRESSION IN NURSING PROFESSIONALS: AN INTEGRATIVE REVIEW

Camila Cabral, Dionathan Carmini, Letícia Rodrigues, Deise de Oliveira Ribeiro, Heitor Biondi

SUMMARY

Objective: This study aims to identify, in national and international literature, scientific evidence associated with the reasons for the high prevalence of depression among nursing workers. **Method:** Integrative literature review, carried out in May 2019, in the LILACS, Medline, Pubmed and Scielo databases, using the descriptors nursing, nurses and depression, without restricting the year. **Results:** The sample consisted of 10 articles, which were published between 1999 and 2016, both national and international. The factors that were most related to the development of depression in nursing professionals were work overload, lack of autonomy, low pay, devaluation of the profession, uncertainty of medical knowledge, lack of resources and job insecurity. **Conclusion:** It has been shown that nursing professionals face numerous difficulties in their daily practice and that factors such as work overload, professional devaluation and poor operating conditions result in professional stress, which can lead to depression and a consequent drop in the quality of care provided to the population.

DESCRIPTORS: Nursing; Depression; Nurses

1. INTRODUCTION

Depression is characterised by persistent sadness and loss of interest in activities previously considered pleasurable, accompanied by cognitive changes that prevent the individual from carrying out daily activities, and the symptoms must persist for at least two weeks to confirm the diagnosis. It is estimated that depression affects around 300 million people worldwide and is therefore an important public health factor to be discussed .[1]

Studies report that the professionals who are most susceptible to a decline in mental health are those who interact most of the time with individuals who need their help, such as nurses, among other professions.[2] Thus, using an integrative literature review, we intend to analyse the prevalence of depression in nursing professionals, given that studies have perceived negative aspects such as anxiety, stress and depression in nursing professionals2,[3] for more than two decades, precisely because it is a profession that deals with various risks in its execution, These include physical, ergonomic, chemical and emotional risks that cause a high level of stress, as well as shift work, job insecurity, professional depreciation, reduced autonomy, long hours spent on bureaucratic tasks,

2 METHOD

which can lead to a feeling of insufficient quality of service and dissatisfaction .[4]

In view of the above, this study aims to identify, in the national and international literature, scientific evidence associated with the reasons for the high prevalence of depression among nursing workers.

This is an integrative literature review, built on the following stages: development of the guiding question; search for primary studies in databases; extraction of data from the studies; evaluation of the selected studies; analysis and synthesis of the results and presentation of the review. The guiding question was: *What evidence is available in the literature about the factors that contribute to depression among nursing professionals?*

The integrative review is a type of review that makes it possible to carry out analyses that go beyond the synthesis of the results of primary studies, encompassing other dimensions of research and which has the potential to develop new theories and research problems, as well as having an international reputation in nursing research and evidence-based practice.[6]

Data was collected in May 2019. To select the articles, the databases Latin American and Caribbean Literature in Health Science (LILACS), Medical Literature Analysis and Retrieval System online (MEDLINE), National Library of Medicine (PubMed) and Scientific Electronic Library Online (Scielo) were consulted. The descriptors (enfermagem, nursing, enfermeiros, nurses, depressão, depression) were combined in different ways to ensure a broad search.

The inclusion criteria for the pre-selection of studies were: studies in English or Portuguese that dealt with depressive disorder. According to the exclusion criteria, articles that were not in the aforementioned languages, those that addressed other mood disorders and those that, after reading in full, did not respond to the objective of this review were excluded.

It is important to emphasise that there was no delimitation in terms of the year the articles were published. The selection was made by carefully reading the titles and abstracts, and the final selection was made of the studies that met the aforementioned inclusion criteria. A full reading of the work was carried out as the final selection criterion for the articles, and those that presented the contributing factors for depression in nurses were selected.

An instrument was used to collect and analyse the data, which was adapted to meet the study's objective. The topics of interest covered in the instrument were: year of publication, country of origin, title, database, study design and sample and associated factors.

In the second stage, the titles and abstracts of the articles were read and analysed from the perspective of the inclusion criteria. In this way, 17 articles were selected. In the third stage, these 17 articles were read in full and 7 were removed because they did not meet the inclusion criteria and did not answer the guiding question of this review, so that the final sample consisted of 10 articles. After establishing the sample, the information to be extracted from the studies was defined and the 10 articles were analysed in depth.

3. RESULTS

This is an integrative review of 10 articles published between 1999 and 2016. Of the sample selected, seven were quantitative and three qualitative, from the following countries: Brazil, China, Japan, Portugal and Turkey. The oldest article dates from 1999 and the most recent from 2016, of which one (10%) was published in 1999, one (10%) in 2005, two (20%) in 2011, four (40%) in 2015 and two (20%) in 2016. It should be noted that at least one of the authors of the studies belongs to a nursing department or school, except for the article *"Stress responses and coping resources in nurses"*, in which the authors are part of the psychology department.

With regard to the population studied in the research, we would highlight nursing professionals aged between 20 and 70, working in public and private hospitals, in cardiology, rehabilitation, internal medicine, intensive care, operating theatres and the emergency department. Nurses working in Basic Health Units with a family health strategy were also part of the sample.

Table 1 - Summary of the studies found, broken down by year of publication, country of origin, title, database, type of study, sample size and factors associated with depression:

Year of publication	Country of origin	Title	Database	Study/sample design	Associated factors
' 1999	Portugal	Stress responses and coping resources in nurses	SciELO	Quantitative study , 62	I Overload labour physical conditions, lack of human/material resources and

				nurses	technicians, excessive number of patients per nurse, lack of privacy , ambiguity of functions, dehumanisation of treatment/ care, risks to their own health, interpersonal conflicts, difficulty in dealing with death, lack of autonomy, lack of opportunities for promotion, hierarchical demands, low pay, responsibility, confli cts, etc. professional, family and social demands, unc ertainty medical knowledge and shift work.
' 2005	Turkey	Effects of Perceived Job Insecurity on Perceived Anxietyand Depressionin Nurses	Pubm ed	Quantitative study , 462 nurses private hospitals	i Having been working for less than a year, insecurity and quantitative and qualitative work, high labour tension and social support
' 2011	Brazil	Prevalence of depression in labour nursing	Scielo	Quantitative study , 67 professional	i Work the night shift, work double shifts and are

		Intensive Care Unit: a study in hospitals in a city in the Algarve north-western São Paulo state		sde nursing	separateor divorced
' 2011	Brazil	Anxiety depression between professionals nursing act as blocks surgical	SciELO	Quantitative study , 221 professionals nursing	i Type of hospital (public/philanthropic or private); Work in more than one health institution (yes or no); and Workload per week (up to 40 hours or more than 40 hours per week).
' 2015	China	Depression, Anxiety and Symptoms of Stress among Hong Kongers Nurses: A Cross-sectional Study	Pubmed	Qualitative study, 850 nurses	i Self-perception of mental health Disagreements with colleagues Sleep disorders Devaluing the profession Stress caused by the environment and personal issues Dissatisfaction work Unpreparedness team Self-doubt

					Lack of leisure time Abs ence of physical exercise
' 2015	Brazil	Depression and suicide risk among prof essionals Nursing: integrative review	SciELO	Integrative Review of Scientific Literature com prising20 articles,	i Environment labour civil, stress, lack of autonomy professional, insecurity in carrying out activities, overload of labour, income family, duty
' 2015	Brazil	Symptomsof depressionand intervening factors among nurses of emergency hospital services	SciELO	Study qualitative, 23 nurses	i Overload workload Excessive working hours, wear and tear, preoccupation with work Unsatisfactory pay Professional devaluation, lack of recognition Lack of working conditions Unprepared staff job insecurity Professional harassment Lack of professional commitment from colleagues Frustration Dissatisfied staff, lack of autonomy for the organisation

					nurse, personal issues, mistrust ageing
' 2015	Japan	Relationships of job demand, job control, and social support on intention to leave and depression sy mptomsin Japanese nurses	Pubm ed	Quantitative study , 1063 nurses	i Demand work, work control, support from supervisors, support from family and friends, working more than 60 hours a week
' 2016	Brazil	Burnoute depressive symptomatology in nurses intensive care: relationship analysis	Scielo	Quantitative study , 91 intensive care nurses	i Income, working hours excessive labour professional fulfilment, emotional exhaustion and depersonalisation
' 2016	Brazil	Work depressive symptomatology in nurses Family Health Strategy	Lilacs	Qualitative study, 59 ESF nurses	i Factors related to number of duties of nurses Overload work Lack of organisational structure and human resources Overcharging Lack of appreciation for nurses

Table 2 - Factors associated with depression in nursing professionals organised into 3 main groups: environmental, personal and operational factors.

Associated factors		
Environmental	**Personal**	**Operational**
Lack of privacy; dehumanisation of treatment/care; risks to their own health; high workload; lack of working conditions; unprepared and rotating staff; job insecurity; harassment professional; lack of professional commitment on the part of colleagues; frustration; team dissatisfied; disagreements with colleagues; stress caused by the environment; interpersonal conflicts at work; working environment; type of hospital (public/philanthropic or private); Work in more than one health institution; lack of promotion opportunities; hierarchical demands; qualitative and quantitative job insecurity; lack of support from supervisors	Poor physical condition; dealing with death; conflict of demands professional, family and social; uncertainty of theoretical knowledge; lack of social support; marital status; support from family and friends; weariness and emotional exhaustion; preoccupation with work; lack of confidence; self-doubt; ageing; self-perception of mental health; sleep disorders; lack of leisure time; lack of physical exercise ; insecurity in developing activities; stress; little professional fulfilment; depersonalisation	Lack of autonomy for nurses; bad technological conditions; human/material resources and technical; excessive number of patients/nurses; work overload; shift work; having been working for less than a year; working the night shift; working double shifts; high work demand; excessive working hours; unsatisfactory remuneration; professional devaluation; job dissatisfaction; high number of activities assigned to nurses. nurses; lack of organisational structure and human resources ; overcharging;

4. DISCUSSION

Although the results of this review indicate that depression in nursing professionals is a condition that has been present for some time, since the oldest article selected for this study was published in 1999, studies show that the prevalence rate of depression is similar to that found in the general population, 3% to 11%[7] The individual who suffers from depression has symptoms that encompass the emotional, cognitive and physical aspects, cognition and the physical, with symptoms such as sadness, decreased pleasure in activities that were previously performed with satisfaction, negative thoughts about oneself, decreased concentration and memory, changes in sleep, appetite and general malaise, as well as a lack of initiative[8] , which can influence the quality of care provided to patients.

In addition, similarities were found between the factors that predispose to this condition in Brazil and in the other countries studied, such as China, Japan, Portugal and Turkey, especially when it comes to high work demand and social support, as shown in *Table 1,* which may indicate that the problems faced by nursing professionals go beyond geographical and cultural barriers, and therefore merit further studies to elucidate this point.

Data obtained in 2017[9] , indicate that there was an 18% increase in the incidence rate of depression in the general population between 2005 and 2015, totalling more than 322 million people worldwide affected by this condition, which mainly affects women; in Brazil, it is estimated that 11.5 million people (5.8% of the population) have depression. It is therefore interesting to analyse the profile of nursing professionals, given that data from 2010[10] showed a total of 1,449,583 nursing professionals in Brazil, 87.24% of whom were women, totalling 1,264,641 female professionals, in order to understand the factors that may predispose this condition in a population that is considered to be more susceptible.

Analysing the results, it was possible to observe the emergence of numerous factors related to the development of depression in nursing professionals. Of these, the most prominent are operational factors such as work overload, lack of autonomy, low pay, devaluation of the profession, lack of resources and job insecurity. In addition to the personal factors, the uncertainty of technical knowledge also appears to be a stressor for nursing professionals. This is in line with the findings of the study *on stress in nurse management*[11] , which associates worker stress with emotional exhaustion, tiredness and situations of high work demand. In addition, specific situations such as relationship problems, double shifts at work and home and pressure from superiors according to the individual's perception are associated with stress[12] , with chronic stress being a predictor of burnout syndrome[13] , a condition that can influence depression[14] , and were consistent with the findings of this integrative review.

The study's limitation was the small sample size of the articles selected, which does not allow for generalisation beyond the population studied. It is therefore important not only to carry out a more in-depth study, but also to implement strategies to reduce the incidence of depression among nursing professionals. In this sense, studies[15] refer to a reduction in working hours, attractive and rewarding working conditions, investment in professional development and social support for teams, including professionals in collective decisions, as some of the measures to prevent stress, burnout and consequently depression.[16]

5. CONCLUSION

Based on the studies analysed in this integrative review, it is clear that nursing professionals suffer from an overload of working hours, undervaluation of the services they provide, interpersonal conflicts at work, as well as a lack of suitable materials in the service environment and unprepared staff, resulting in professional stress. Another relevant factor that was also found to be common in the aforementioned studies was unsatisfactory pay, often leading to a lack of time for leisure because workers need to work long hours.

In fact, these contributors influence depression, since the environment has a strong influence on this, which makes the professional vulnerable. It should be emphasised that these factors interfere with the services provided to the population, which is why it is so important for professionals to rotate and for them to be psychologically monitored, and for them to be understood not just as health workers, but as human beings who also need care for their own health .

The articles used for this integrative review aim to highlight the importance of this care and attention to the factors that influence depression so that there can be changes and a decrease in the growing number of nursing professionals diagnosed with depression.

REFERENCES

1 Pan American Health Organisation. **Depression: what you need to know.** 2016-2017. Disponívelem: <https://www.paho.org/bra/index.php?option=com_content&view=article&id=5372:depressao-o-what-you-need-to-know&Itemid=822> Accessed: 20 May 2019

2. Baba, V. Vishwanath. Galperin, L. Bella. Lituchy, R. Terri. **Occupational mental health: a study of work-related depression among nurses in the Caribbean**. International Journal of Nursing Studies Volume 36, Issue 2, April 1999, Pages163-169 . Availableat : <https://www.sciencedirect.com/science/article/abs/pii/S0020748999000024> Accessed on : 20 May 2019

3. FRANCO, Gianfábio Pimentel; BARROS, Alba Lucia Botura Leite de and NOGUEIRA-MARTINS, Luiz Antonio. **Quality of life and depressive symptoms in nursing residents**. Rev. Latino-Am. Enfermagem [online]. 2005, vol.13, n.2, pp.139-144. Available at: <http://www.scielo.br/scielo.php?pid=S0104-11692005000200002&script=sci_abstract&tlng=en> Accessed: 20 May 2019

4. ARAÚJO, G.S et al. **Profile of nursing workers accompanied by a multiprofessional mental health team**. Revista Rene, v.15, n.2, p. 257-63. 2014. Available at: <http://www.redalyc.org/html/3240/324031263010/index.html> Accessed: 25 May 2019

5. Barbosa, Khivia Kiss Silva; Vieira, Kay Francis Leal; Alves, Estela Rodrigues Paiva; Virgínio, Nereide Andrade. **DEPRESSIVE SYMPTOMS AND SUICIDAL IDEATION IN HOSPITAL NURSES AND DOCTORS.** Available at: <https://periodicos.ufsm.br/reufsm/article/view/5910/pdf> Accessed on: 25 May 2019

6. Soares, Cassia; Hoga, Luiza; Peduzzi, Marina; Sangaleti, Carine; Yonekura, Tatiana; Silva, Deborah. **Integrative review: concepts and methods used in nursing.** Rev. Esc Enferm USP 2014; 48(2):335-45. Available at: <http://www.scielo.br/pdf/reeusp/v48n2/pt_0080-6234-reeusp-48-02-335.pdf> Accessed on: 20 May 2019

7. Rios, Kátia Assalvi; Barbosa, Dulce Aparecida; Belasco, Angélica Gonçalves. **Evaluation of the quality of life and depression of nursing technicians and assistants.** Rev. Latino-Am. Enfermagem[online]. 2010, vol.18, n.3, pp.413- 420 Available at:<http://www.scielo.br/scielo.php?pid=S0104-11692010000300017&script=sci_abstract&tlng=en> Accessed: 21 May 2019

8. Atkison, R. L., Atkinson, R. C., Smith, E. E., Dary, B. J., Nolen-Hoeksema, S., Smith, C. Hilgard's Introduction to Psychology. Translation by Daniel Bueno. (13ª ed.). Porto Alegre: Artmed, 2002. apud Pacheco, Ana Carolina. **Anxiety, depression, stress, coping strategies and social support in nurses who work shifts and fixed daytime hours**. Lusófona Scientific Repository. Portugal, 2013. Availableat : <http://recil.grupolusofona.pt/handle/10437/4996> Accessed: 21 May 2019

9. United Nations Brazil. **WHO records increase in cases of depression worldwide**. 2017. Available at: <https://nacoesunidas.org/oms-registra- increase-of-cases-of-depression-all-over-the-world-in-brazil-are-115-million-people/> Accessed on: 21 May 2019

10. Federal Nursing Council (Cofen). **Analysing data from nursing professionals in the Regional Councils.** 2011. Available at:<www.cofen.gov.br/wp-content/uploads/2012/03/researchprofessionals.pdf> Accessed: 23 May 2019

11. Lautert L, Chaves EHB, Moura GSS. **Stress in the managerial activity of nurses**. Revista Panam Salud Publica 1999; 6(6):415-25. Available at: <https://scielosp.org/pdf/rpsp/1999.v6n6/415-425/pt> Accessed on: 23 May 2019

12. STACCIARINI, Jeanne Marie R. and TROCCOLI, Bartholomeu T.. **Stress in the occupational activity of nurses.** Rev. Latino-Am.

Enfermagem [online]. 2001, vol.9, n.2, pp.17-25. Available at: <http://www.scielo.br/scielo.php?pid=S0104-11692001000200003&script=sci_abstract&tlng=en> Accessed: 23 May 2019

13. RIBEIRO, Samara dos Santos; MOTTA, Elizângela Araujo Pestana. **ASSOCIATION BETWEEN BURNOUT SYNDROME AND CORTISOL HORMONE**. Rev. Ciênc. Saúde v.16, n. 2, p. 87-93, jul-dez, 2014. Available at: <http://www.periodicoseletronicos.ufma.br/index.php/rcisaude/issue/view/285> Accessed on: 23 May 2019

14. Murcho, Nuno Álvaro C; de Jesus, Saul Neves; Pacheco, José Eusébio Palma. **The relationship between depression at work and burnout: An empirical study with nurses.** Psic., Saúde & Doenças v.11 n.1 Lisboa 2010. Disponívelem : <http://www.scielo.mec.pt/scielo.php?script=sci_arttext&pid=S1645-00862010000100003> Accessed: 24 May 2019

15. PINTO, A. **Burnout versus stress: investigations in professionals**. 2008. Nursing. Ano 20, n° 240, p. 6-10. *apud* Pereira, Telmo; Oliveira, Vanessa. **Anxiety, depression and burnout in nurses - Impact of shift work.** Revista de Enfermagem Referência - III - n.º 7 - 2012. Available at: <http://www.scielo.mec.pt/scielo.php?script=sciarttext&pid=S0874-02832012000200005> Accessed on: 25 May 2019

16. Mcintyre, Teresa Mendonça; Mcintyre, Scott Elmes; Silvério, Jorge. **Stress responses and coping resources in nurses.** Psychological Analysis (1999), 3 (XVII): 513-527. Available at: <http://www.scielo.mec.pt/pdf/aps/v17n3/v17n3a08.pdf> Accessed: 20 May 2019

17. Boya FO, Demiral Y, Ergor A, Akvardar Y, De Witte H. **Effects of perceived job insecurity on perceived anxiety and depression in nurses**. Ind Health. 2008Dec ;46(6):613-9. Available at : <https://www.ncbi.nlm.nih.gov/pubmed/19088414> Accessed: 20 May 2019

18. Dias, Ana Paula Vieira; Vargas, Divane de. **Prevalence of depression in Intensive Care Unit nursing workers: a study in hospitals in a city in the north-west of the state of São Paulo**. Rev. Latino-Am. Enfermagem 19(5):[09 screens] Sep.-Oct. 2011. Available

at: <http://www.scielo.br/pdf/rlae/v19n5/pt 08.pdf> Accessed on: 20 May 2019

19. Schmidt, Denise Rodrigues Costa; Dantas, Rosana Aparecida Spadoti; Marziale, Maria Helena Palucci. **Anxiety and depression among nursing professionals working in operating theatres.** Rev. esc. enferm. USP vol.45 no.2 São Paulo Apr. 2011. Available at: <http://www.scielo.br/scielo.php?script=sciarttext&pid=S0080- 62342011000200026> Accessed on: 21 May 2019.

20. Cheung T; Yip PS. **Depression, Anxiety and Symptoms of Stress among Hong Kong Nurses: A Cross-sectional Study. Int J Environ Res Public Health.** 2015 Sep 7; 12(9): 11072-100. Available at: <https://www.ncbi.nlm.nih.gov/pubmed/26371020> Accessed on: 21 May 2019

21. Silva, Darlan dos Santos; Tavares, Natália Vieira da Silva; Alexandre, Alícia Regina Gomes; Freitas, Daniel Antunes; Brêda, Mércia Zeviani; Albuquerque, Maria Cícera dos Santos; Neto, Valfrido Leão de Melo. **Depression and suicide risk among nursing professionals: an integrative review.** Rev Esc Enferm USP -2015 ; 49(6): 1027-1036. Available at: <http://www.scielo.br/pdf/reeusp/v49n6/pt 0080-6234-reeusp-49-06-1027.pdf> Accessed: 21 May 2019.

22. Oliveira, Felipe Perucci; Mazzaia, Maria Cristina;de Oliveira, Felipe Perucci. **Symptoms of depression and intervening factors among nurses of emergency hospital services. Acta paul.** enferm. vol.28 no.3 São Paulo May/June 2015. Available at: <http://www.scielo.br/scielo.php?pid=S0103-21002015000300209&script=sciarttext&tlng=en> Accessed on: 21 May 2019

23. Saijo, Yasuaki; Yoshioka, Eiji; Kawanishi, Yasuyuki; Nakagi, Yoshihiko; Itoh, Toshihiro; Yoshida, Takahiko. **Relationships of job demand, job control, and social support on intention to leave and depressive symptoms in Japanese nurses.** Ind Health. 2016 Jan; 54(1): 32-41. Available at: <https://www.ncbi.nlm.nih.gov/pmc/articles/PMC4791291> Accessed on: 21 May 2019

24. Vasconcelos EM, De Martino MMF, França SPS. **Burnout and depressive symptoms in intensive care nurses: relationship analysis.** Rev Bras Enferm [Internet]. 2018;71(1):135-41. Available in : <http://www.scielo.br/pdf/reben/v71n1/pt 0034-7167-reben-71-01-0135.pdf>

Access : 22 May of 2019.

25. Fernandes, Daniella Marques; Marcolan, João Fernando. **Work and depressive symptomatology in Family Health Strategy nurses.** SMAD, Rev. Eletrônica Saúde

Mental Álcool Drog. (Ed. port.) vol.13 no.1 Ribeirão Preto, 2017. Available at: <http://pepsic.bvsalud.org/scielo.php?script=sciarttext&pid=S1806-69762017000100006&lng=en&nrm=iso&tlng=en> Accessed: 22 May 2019.

5.CEREBRAL BLOOD FLOW VERSUS ASPIRATION OF SECRETIONS AND ITS POSSIBLE COMPLICATIONS/INJURIES IN NEONATOLOGY.

Leandro Corrêa, Mônica Carvalho Sanchez Stopiglia, Jeferson Ventura

SUMMARY

Advances in neonatal care in recent decades have been responsible for a significant reduction in mortality rates among high-risk newborns. Physiotherapy in Neonatal Intensive Care Units can contribute to injury prevention when it is based on knowledge of the particularities, the pathophysiology of the disease, the physiology of cerebral blood flow, physiotherapy techniques and the direct and indirect relationship of the procedures performed with cerebral haemodynamics. The haemodynamic and gas exchange disorders resulting from endotracheal aspiration imply changes in cerebral blood flow that can lead to the development of serious neurological morbidities, such as periventricular leukomalacia and periventricular-intraventricular haemorrhage. Airway suction is a procedure often used in neonatal intensive care units to maintain airway patency, especially in patients with ineffective coughing, such as newborns. This is because the accumulation of secretions is inevitable in these patients. Although it seems like a simple procedure, care must be taken to avoid undesirable effects. These effects include adverse cardiovascular effects, alterations to the autonomic nervous system and an increase in cerebral blood flow and intracranial pressure. Few studies have investigated the influence of respiratory physiotherapy on brain damage or changes in cerebral blood flow in newborns, but some considerations can be made based on the physiological principles of secretion aspiration.

Keywords: newborns, respiratory physiotherapy, airway aspiration.

1 INTRODUCTION

Nowadays, children with low gestational age are identified much more frequently than in the last 30 years in neonatal intensive care units (NICUs), and high rates of mortality and morbidity caused by brain injuries are reported in this population (VAN, JAEGERE, RIMENSBERGER, 2013).

Medical progress and advances in neonatal care have resulted in longer survival for increasingly premature newborns (NBs). However, prolonged NICU care is associated with an increased incidence of permanent deficits in neuropsychosensory-motor development among survivors.

Respiratory physiotherapy has been an effective resource in the prevention and treatment of various lung diseases, especially for the removal of bronchial secretion.

In the NICU, neonatal physiotherapy consists of procedures carried out by the physiotherapist in the period between the clamping of the umbilical cord and 28 days after birth, which include handling the motor and pulmonary parts of the NB (ABREU; 2003, 2006).

The control of cerebral blood flow (CBF) involves complex neural and metabolic mechanisms, which are still immature in the pre-term newborn (PTNB).

Changes in CBF are often associated with upper airway obstruction, severe respiratory diseases, intermittent positive pressure ventilation, tracheal aspiration and circulatory volume expansion (MARBA ST, ARANHA NETTO; 2002. P. 289 - 98).

As we have seen, the vast majority of situations that have been shown to cause significant changes in CBF in term newborns and PTNBs are related to respiratory dysfunctions, which lead to the need for a longer period of hospitalisation and ventilatory support and, consequently, a greater risk of complications associated with mechanical ventilation and its procedures.

One method used in Intensive Care Centres is Invasive Mechanical Ventilation (IMV). However, its use predisposes patients to risks such as tracheal injury, barotrauma and oxygen toxicity. In addition to these factors, patients undergoing IMV are prone to respiratory problems due to ineffective coughing, predisposing to the accumulation of secretions (JUDSON, 1994).

Various physiotherapeutic manoeuvres are being evaluated for their effectiveness in removing secretions from the respiratory tract and the risk of adverse effects, but more clinical studies are still needed to prove their effectiveness.

Tracheal aspiration, widely used to remove secretions from the upper and lower airways, carries a risk of adverse effects such as bradycardia and hypoxaemia (HADDAS, 2006).

Although the benefits of aspiration for removing secretions from the airways are clear in clinical practice, the side effects associated with it have never been studied or, above all, evaluated (STILLER, 2000).

Cerebrovascular lesions, such as Periventricular Intraventricular Haemorrhage (PIVH) and Periventricular Leukomalacia (PVL), are the main causes of neurodevelopmental changes (ARGYROPOULOU MI, 2010).

Recent studies have described new types of diffuse lesions in the white and grey matter in newborns submitted to long periods of mechanical ventilation. Ventilatory assistance is one of the main supports offered in the treatment of various diseases in NB.

Few studies have investigated the influence of respiratory physiotherapy on brain injuries in newborns in terms of changes in CBF, so there is a lack of studies to recognise the physiology of CBF control in newborns, identifying the procedures that promote changes in CBF, as well as the risk of neurological injuries.

The aim of endotracheal suction is to ensure the patency of the airway necessary to facilitate ventilation and prevent complications related to secretion accumulation. However, there are complications associated with this procedure.

2 METHODOLOGY

The methodology of this study is a bibliographical review that carried out a systematic search of the literature and content analysis, with the aim of analysing changes in cerebral blood flow through the procedure of secretion aspiration.

The main sources for this research were consultations of study databases such as academic journals, websites, digital libraries, scientific articles and books on the subject published over the last thirty years.

According to Cervo, Bervian and da Silva (2007, p.61), bibliographical research "is the basic procedure for monographic studies, through which we seek to master the state of the art on a given topic".

To select the articles, we first read the abstracts, checking that they contained information that met the following criteria: crossing the descriptors with newborn or neonate, preterm, neonatal respiratory physiotherapy, cerebral blood flow, secretion aspiration.

Very limited articles and other studies on the subject were identified, and the decision was made to use those that came closest to the object under study. The final selection of materials was read in full for the purposes of this work.

3 RESULTS

The main objectives of respiratory physiotherapy are to prevent and reduce the consequences of bronchial obstruction by secretion, such as hyperinflation, atelectasis, changes in the ventilation-perfusion ratio and increased respiratory work (KAISER JR, GAUS CH, PONT MM, WILLIAMS DK, 2004;26:279-85).

The adverse effects of endotracheal suction directly related to the CNS include an increase in ICP, an increase in cerebral blood volume related to changes in CO2 tension, and a decrease in cerebral oxygenation due to a decrease in oxygen supply (AARC GUIDELINES FOR CLINICAL PRACTICE, 2010). The aspiration procedure has been associated with a transient decrease in heart rate, as a parasympathetic reflex to the discharge of pulmonary pressure receptors. On the other hand, sympathetic activation is due to transient hypoxaemia and direct tactile stimulation of the sympathetic receptors in the trachea, triggering systemic arterial hypertension (LIMPEROPOLOUS, et al, 2008).

The endotracheal suction procedure is necessary. Despite this, it is associated with a number of transient disturbances in haemodynamic stability, and impaired gas exchange leads to a regulation of cerebral blood flow and the subsequent development of neonatal brain damage (YOUNG CS. 1984).

When properly indicated and carried out, secretion aspiration is of great value in the treatment of patients who are unable to expel their secretions spontaneously, providing them with post-procedure respiratory relief and comfort.

However, the method of aspiration causes not only physiological changes, but also neurobehavioural ones that can have dangerous consequences for the NB.

The professionals involved in the day-to-day running of the NICU must be committed to reducing the damage that aspiration can cause to the NB's neuropsychomotor development.

In this context, knowledge about the behaviour of the NB's CSF during respiratory physiotherapy can contribute to safer physiotherapeutic care, especially during the first few weeks of life.

In general, contraindications to secretion aspiration are related to the possibility of the patient experiencing adverse reactions or a worsening of the clinical condition as a result of the procedure.

The endotracheal suction procedure alone does not bring benefits to the patient, and it is important to note that secretions present in the peripheral airways are not removed with this technique alone; therefore, the assessment of the timing of suction must be individualised (GONÇALVES RL; TSUZUKI LM; CARVALHO, MG; 2015).

The physiotherapist must conduct the dynamics of the therapy according to the specific assessment and identification of the needs of the clinical condition presented by each patient.

4 DISCUSSION

One question that needs to be explained is whether respiratory physiotherapy, in an attempt to improve lung function, causes changes in CBF that are harmful to small newborns.

Few studies have reported quantitatively on the pattern of cerebral haemodynamic behaviour in this population before, during and after the secretion aspiration procedure.

Cerebral flow immediately after birth largely reflects the circulatory adaptations that follow the neonatal period (VOLPE, 1995). This flow changes significantly in the first 24 hours of life (DEEG & RUPRECHT, 1989).

In newborns, alterations in CBF can cause rupture of the fragile capillary vessels of the germinal matrix, leading to peri- or intraventricular haemorrhage.

Practice often shows us that more and more PTNB have respiratory diseases, and physiotherapy is one of the treatments in the NICU.

IVH is a highly prevalent problem in newborns, since the most common place of origin for bleeding is the germinal matrix (MG), which only begins to evolve around the 34th gestational week[a] when the cortical migration process ends and practically disappears completely around the 36th gestational week (ARANHA NETTO A,1998).

IVH is mainly due to the increase in CBF in the immature microvasculature of the MG. Some authors state that the period of greatest risk for IVH is the first week of life, when 90% of haemorrhages are diagnosed in their most complete form (BUCKLEY, COOK, DURDURAN T, KIM MN, ZHOU C, CHOE R, 2009).

Various factors can contribute to the rupture of the germinal matrix vessels. The risk factors for IVH include pre- and post-natal factors, maternal and obstetric factors and factors intrinsic to the NB. Some sources of risk are: infection, maternal inflammation, severe respiratory distress, need for mechanical ventilation, endotracheal suction, vigorous resuscitation, hypoxaemia, acidosis, pneumothorax and convulsions.

LPV should also be mentioned, which in general is an ischaemic complication, with necrosis of the white matter, particularly in the regions adjacent to the external angles of the lateral ventricles.

Risk factors include neonatal events capable of causing cerebral ischaemia such as severe hypotension, hypocapnia, PDA with retrograde diastolic flow and severe respiratory diseases requiring extracorporeal membrane oxygenation, apnoea with hypoxia and bradycardia.

PVL is a brain injury that is often associated with permanent neurological sequelae and is currently one of the main causes of cerebral palsy. The severity of the sequelae depends on the extent of the injury. The most frequent sequelae observed are motor dysfunctions, particularly spastic diplegia, in which the lower limbs are more affected (COWAN F, WHITELAW A, WERTHEIM D, SILVERMAN M. 1991;66).

Even with the application of good practices in neonatal care, there are still sequelae and dysfunctions in the evolution of these newborns and a variety of neurodevelopmental problems.

Some studies have investigated the influence of respiratory physiotherapy on brain damage in newborns.

According to Harding et al. (1998), in an attempt to discover the possible causes of the increase in the incidence of this brain injury, they observed an association between encephaloclastic porencephaly and hypotension, birth with non-cephalic presentation and respiratory physiotherapy.

The increase in CBF velocity and cerebral blood volume seem to remain high for 25 minutes after the endotracheal suction procedure and are directly related to the increase in $PaCO^2$, while PaO2 does not seem to have a significant influence on CBF (AARC GUIDELINES FOR CLINICAL PRACTICE, 2010).

In endotracheal aspiration, changes in mean arterial pressure can also affect CBF, especially in NB who have limited cerebral autoregulation, with little influence in NB with full autoregulation (EVANS, SYDDALL, BUTT, KINNEY, 2014).

There is still no common understanding in the literature about how open or closed suction systems can affect the cerebral repercussions of suction. These results have generated a great deal of controversy and, as a result, new research on this subject is currently being carried out.

5 CONCLUSION

The haemodynamic and gas exchange disorders resulting from endotracheal aspiration imply changes in CBF that can lead to the development of serious neurological morbidities such as PVL and IVH.

According to the findings, it can be concluded that the tracheal aspiration technique brings about important changes in the vital data of neonates, such as: increased blood pressure, bradycardia, decreased lung compliance. This is reflected in the brain through vasodilation and deoxygenation.

Considering that patients undergoing mechanical ventilation may require endotracheal suction to maintain airway patency, there can be no absolute contraindication to the procedure.

However, care must be taken when choosing when to carry out the procedure, as it should only be carried out when there is an indication and not routinely.

Although there are studies evaluating the relationship between respiratory physiotherapy and the occurrence of brain damage, no study to date has presented quantitative assessments of CBF in NBs before, during and after respiratory physiotherapy manoeuvres.

BIBLIOGRAPHICAL REFERENCES

AARC CLINICAL PRACTICE GUIDELINES. **Endotracheal suctioning on mechanically ventilated patients with artificial airways.** 2010. Respiratory Care. June; 55(6); 758-764.

ARANHA NETTO A. **Cerebral blood flow velocity by doppler ultrasound on the first day of life of polycythaemic newborns** [Doctoral Thesis] Campinas (SP): Universidade Estadual de Campinas ;1998.

BUCKLEY EM, COOK NM, DURDURAN T, KIM MN, ZHOU C, CHOE R, **et al. Cerebral haemodynamics in preterm intants during positional intervention measured with**

COWAN F, WHITELAW A, WERTHEIM D, SILVERMAN M. **Cerebral blood flow velocity changes after rapid administration of surfactant.** Arch Dis Child 1991;66(10specNo):1105-9. Available at : , www.ncbi.nlm.nih.gov/pubmed/1750756. Accessed 07 January 2019.

EVANS, J; SYDDALL S; BUTT W; KINNEY, S. **Comparison of open and closed suction os safety, efficacy and nursing time in a paediatric care unit.** Australian Critical care. 2014; 27; 70-74. Available at: , www.ncbi.nlm.nih.gov/pubmed/24636425. Accessed on 10 February 2019.

GONÇALVES RL; TSUZUKI LM; CARVALHO, MG. **Endotracheal suction in intubated newborns: an integrative literature review.** Ver Bra Ter Intensiva. 2015: 27 (3): 284-292

GUZMAN EA, BERTAGNON JRD, JULIANO Y. **Frequency of periintraventricular haemorrhage and its associated factors in preterm newborns.** Einsten. 2010; 8 (3 pt 1): 315-9. Available at: http://www.scielo.br/scielo.php?pid=S1679-45082010000300315&script=sciarttext&tlng=en. Accessed on 02 February 2019.

HADDAD, Eliane Rezende; COSTA, Larissa Cristina Dias da; NEGRINI, Fernanda; SAMPAIO, Luciana Maria Melosa;, **Physiotherapeutic approaches for the removal of airway secretions in newborns.** *Pediatria* (São Paulo) 2006; 28(2): 135-0. Available at: http://www.scielo.br/scielo.php?script=scinlinks&ref=000078&pid=S0103-51502011000100008000048lng=pt. Accessed on 10 January 2019.

HARDING JE, MILES FKI, BECROFT DMO, ALLEN BC, KNIGHT DB. **Chest physiotherapy may be associated with brain damage in extremely premature infants.** J Pediatr 1998;132:440-4. Available at: www.ncbi.nlm.nih.qov/pubmed/9544898. Accessed on 25 March 2019.

KAISER JR, GAUS CH, PONT MM, WILLIAMS DK. **Hypercapnia during the first 3 days of life is associated with severe intraventricular haemorrhage in very low birth weight infants.** J Perinatol 2004;26:279-85. Available at: www.ncbi.nlm.nih.qov/pubmed/16554847. Accessed 21 March 2019.

LIMPEROPOULOS C. et al. **Cerebral haemodynamic changes during intensive care of preterm infants.** Pediatrics. 2008; 122(5):e1006-13. Available at:

www.ncbi.nlm.nih.qov/pubmed/18931348. Accessed on 13 February 2019.

MARBA ST, ARANHA NETTO A. **Use of Doppler flowmetry in transfontanellar cranial ultrasound.** In: Alves Filho N, T rindade Filho O, Fiori RM, editors. Clinical Perinatology. Rio de Janeiro: Medsi; 2002. p. 289 - 98. Available at: http://www.scielo.br/scielo.php?pid=S0103-05822016000200178&script=sciarttext&tlnq=pt. Accessed on 08 February 2019.

NICOLAU CM, FALCÃO MC. **Effects of respiratory physiotherapy in newborns: a critical analysis of the literature.** Rev. Paul Pediatra. 2007;25:72-5.

NICOLAU CM, LAHÓZ AL. **Respiratory physiotherapy in paediatric and neonatal intensive care: an evidence-based review.** Paediatrics (SP) 2007; 29(3): 216-221.

VAN KAAN AH; DE JAEGERE AP; RIMENSBERGER PC. **Incidence of hypo- and hyper-capnia in a cross-sectional European cohort of ventilated newborn infants.** Arch Dis Child Fetal Neonatal Ed. 2013; 98: F323- F326. Available at: www.ncbi.nlm.nih.qov/pubmed/23241364. Accessed 16 February 2019.

YOUNG CS. **A review of the adverse effects of airway suction.**
Physiotherapy 1984; 70(3): 104-108.

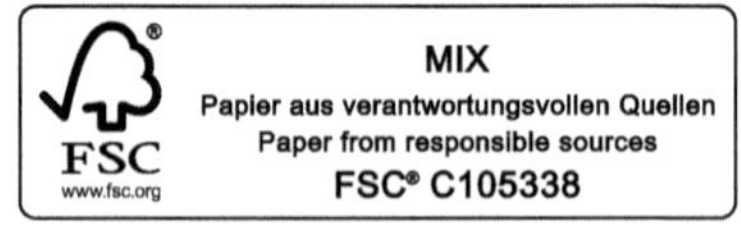

Printed by Books on Demand GmbH, Norderstedt / Germany